Holistic Natural Remedies
for Anxiety and Stress

Jane Evans

Table of Contents

Preface

A New Approach to Healing

In this era of unprecedented challenges and uncertainty, anxiety and stress have become pervasive companions in our lives. The relentless demands of modern society, coupled with a constant bombardment of negative news and information, have taken a toll on our collective mental and emotional well-being.

Conventional approaches to managing anxiety and stress, such as medication and therapy, while helpful in certain cases, often fall short in addressing the root causes of these conditions. Medications may provide temporary relief, but they often come with a host of side effects and do not promote lasting inner peace. Therapy, while valuable for exploring the psychological underpinnings of anxiety and stress, can be time-consuming and expensive.

This guide offers a fresh perspective on healing anxiety and stress, guiding readers towards a holistic and natural approach that promotes lasting inner peace and well-being. Rooted in the wisdom of ancient traditions and the latest scientific research, this book

provides a roadmap for transforming
our relationship with stress and anxiety,
empowering us to cultivate resilience
and inner harmony.

The Holistic Paradigm

Holistic healing recognizes that mind,
body, and spirit are interconnected and
interdependent. It seeks to address the
whole person, rather than focusing
solely on symptoms. This approach
acknowledges that anxiety and stress are
not merely psychological conditions,
but rather manifestations of imbalances
within our entire being.

By adopting a holistic approach, we can
uncover the underlying causes of our
anxiety and stress, whether they be
physical, emotional, mental, or spiritual.
This deeper understanding allows us to
develop personalized strategies for

healing that addresses our unique needs and circumstances.

For instance, if we are experiencing anxiety due to poor sleep, a holistic approach would not only address the symptoms of anxiety but also explore the root causes of our sleep disturbances. This may involve examining our sleep habits, identifying any underlying medical conditions, and making lifestyle changes to promote better sleep hygiene.

The Power of Nature

Nature offers a wealth of resources for healing anxiety and stress. From calming herbs to soothing scents and nourishing foods, the natural world provides us with a gentle and effective means of restoring balance and tranquility to our lives.

This book explores the therapeutic benefits of a variety of natural remedies, including:

Herbal remedies: Discover the calming and anxiolytic properties of herbs such as chamomile, lavender, and valerian root. Learn how to prepare and use herbal teas, tinctures, and essential oils to promote relaxation and reduce stress.

Aromatherapy: Explore the power of scent to influence mood and create a sense of calm. Discover how essential oils can be used in diffusers, baths, and massage to promote relaxation and reduce anxiety.

Healing through nutrition: Learn how diet can play a significant role in managing anxiety and stress. Discover which foods to embrace and which to avoid, and gain practical tips for creating a nourishing and anxiety-reducing diet.

Mind-Body Practices

Mind-body practices, such as mindfulness and meditation, have been shown to be highly effective in reducing anxiety and stress. These practices help us to cultivate inner peace, regulate our emotions, and develop greater resilience to stress.

This book provides detailed guidance on a variety of mind-body practices, including:

Mindfulness: Learn how to bring your attention to the present moment, without judgment. Discover how mindfulness can help you to observe your thoughts and feelings without getting caught up in them, reducing anxiety and promoting inner calm.

Meditation: Explore different meditation techniques, including guided meditations, breathwork, and mantra meditation. Learn how to use meditation to cultivate inner peace, reduce stress, and connect with your inner wisdom.

Yoga and Tai Chi: Discover the mind and body benefits of yoga and tai chi, which combine gentle physical movements with mindfulness and breathing techniques. Learn how these practices can promote relaxation, reduce stress, and improve overall well-being.

Creating a Tranquil Environment

Our surroundings can have a profound impact on our emotional well-being. By creating a tranquil and supportive environment, we can reduce external stressors and cultivate a sense of inner peace.

This book provides practical tips for creating a tranquil environment, including:

Decluttering and organizing: Discover how a cluttered and disorganized environment can contribute to stress and anxiety. Learn how to declutter your home and workplace, creating a more serene and calming space.

Surrounding yourself with nature: Learn how spending time in nature can reduce stress and promote relaxation. Discover how to incorporate natural elements into your home and workplace, such as plants, natural light, and soothing colors.

Creating a relaxing sanctuary: Learn how to create a dedicated space in your home or workplace where you can retreat for relaxation and stress relief. Discover the importance of comfortable seating, calming décor, and soft lighting in creating a tranquil sanctuary.

Embracing Self-Care

Self-care is essential for maintaining our mental and emotional well-being. When we prioritize self-care, we are better able to cope with stress and anxiety and cultivate inner peace.

This book provides practical tips for incorporating self-care into your daily routine, including:

Getting enough sleep: Discover the vital role of sleep in reducing anxiety and stress. Learn how to create a relaxing bedtime routine and establish healthy sleep habits.

Exercising regularly: Explore the mood-boosting and stress-reducing benefits of exercise. Discover different types of exercise that can help to reduce anxiety and promote relaxation.

Spending time with loved ones: Learn the importance of social connection in reducing anxiety and stress. Discover how to nurture relationships with family and friends, and how to build a strong support system.

Practicing gratitude: Explore the transformative power of gratitude in reducing anxiety and promoting well-being. Learn how to incorporate gratitude practices into your daily routine, such as keeping a gratitude journal or practicing mindful appreciation.

Embracing Change and Growth

Life is inherently dynamic, and change is an integral part of the human experience. While change can be challenging, it also presents opportunities for growth and transformation.

This book emphasizes the importance of embracing change and growth, and provides tools and strategies for navigating life's transitions with greater ease and resilience. Readers will learn how to:

Identify and challenge negative thought patterns: Discover how negative thought patterns can contribute to anxiety and stress. Learn how to identify and challenge these patterns, and develop more positive and realistic ways of thinking.

Cultivate resilience: Explore the concept of resilience and its importance in managing anxiety and stress. Learn how to develop coping mechanisms, build inner strength, and bounce back from adversity.

Find meaning and purpose: Discover the power of meaning and purpose in reducing anxiety and promoting well-being. Learn how to identify your values, set goals, and live a life that is aligned with your authentic self.

Conclusion: Finding Your Path to Serenity

This book is an invitation to embark on a journey towards inner peace and well-being. By adopting a holistic approach to healing anxiety and stress, readers can uncover the root causes of these conditions and develop personalized strategies for lasting transformation.

The path to serenity is unique for each individual, and this book provides a wealth of tools and resources to support readers on their journey. Whether you are struggling with mild anxiety or chronic stress, this guide will empower you with the knowledge and tools you need to cultivate inner peace, reduce stress, and live a more fulfilling life.

Chapter 1

Understanding Anxiety and Stress

Anxiety and stress are normal human emotions that everyone experiences from time to time. However, when these emotions become excessive or chronic, they can interfere with our daily lives and overall well-being.

Anxiety is a feeling of nervousness, worry, or unease, typically about an imminent event or something with an uncertain outcome. It is often accompanied by physical symptoms such as sweating, trembling, and shortness of breath.

Stress is a state of mental or emotional strain or tension resulting from adverse or demanding circumstances. It can be caused by a variety of factors, including work, relationships, finances, and major life events.

Types of Anxiety Disorders

Anxiety disorders are a group of mental health conditions characterized by excessive fear or anxiety. Some common types of anxiety disorders include:

Generalized anxiety disorder (GAD): Persistent and excessive anxiety and worry about a variety of topics, even when there is no obvious trigger.

Panic disorder: Sudden and unexpected panic attacks, which are characterized by intense fear and physical symptoms such as chest pain, shortness of breath, and dizziness.

Social anxiety disorder (SAD): Intense fear of being judged or embarrassed in social situations.

Phobias: Intense fear of specific objects or situations, such as spiders, heights, or flying.

Obsessive-compulsive disorder (OCD): Unwanted and intrusive thoughts (obsessions) that lead to repetitive behaviors (compulsions).

Types of Stress

Stress can be classified into two main types:

Acute stress: is a short-term response to a specific stressor, such as a job interview or a car accident. It typically causes a "fight-or-flight" response, which prepares the body to respond to danger.

Chronic stress: is long-term stress that can be caused by ongoing problems, such as financial difficulties, relationship problems, or work overload. Chronic stress can have a negative impact on both physical and mental health.

Causes of Anxiety and Stress

Anxiety and stress can be caused by a variety of factors, including:

Genetic factors: Some people are more likely to experience anxiety and stress due to their genes.

Personality traits: People who are more prone to negative thinking, perfectionism, and avoidance are more likely to experience anxiety and stress.

Life experiences: Traumatic or stressful life experiences, such as childhood abuse or neglect, can increase the risk of developing anxiety and stress disorders.

Medical conditions: Some medical conditions, such as thyroid problems and heart disease, can cause anxiety and stress.

Substance use: Alcohol and drug use can worsen anxiety and stress.

Symptoms of Anxiety and Stress

Anxiety and stress can cause a wide range of physical, emotional, and cognitive symptoms, including:

Physical symptoms: sweating, trembling, shortness of breath, heart palpitations, muscle tension, headaches, stomach aches, and nausea.

Emotional symptoms: irritability, anger, sadness, nervousness, worry, fear, and panic.

Cognitive symptoms: difficulty concentrating, forgetfulness, racing thoughts, nightmares, and intrusive thoughts

Impact of Anxiety and Stress

Anxiety and stress can have a significant impact on our lives, including:

Physical health: Anxiety and stress can weaken the immune system, increase the risk of chronic diseases, and worsen existing health conditions.

Mental health: Anxiety and stress can lead to depression, insomnia, and other mental health problems.

Relationships: Anxiety and stress can strain relationships with family, friends, and romantic partners.

Work and school: Anxiety and stress can interfere with work and school performance, leading to absenteeism, decreased productivity, and difficulty concentrating.

Quality of life: Anxiety and stress can reduce overall quality of life, making it difficult to enjoy activities and relationships.

If you are experiencing anxiety or stress that is interfering with your daily life, it is important to seek professional help. A therapist can help you to identify the root causes of your anxiety and stress, develop coping mechanisms, and create a plan for healing.

Chapter 2

The Connection Between Mind and Body

The mind and body are inextricably linked, and what affects one inevitably affects the other. This connection is evident in the way that stress, anxiety, and other mental health conditions can manifest as physical symptoms, such as headaches, stomach aches, and fatigue. Conversely, physical health problems can also lead to mental health issues, such as depression and anxiety.

The Gut-Brain Axis

One of the most important pathways through which the mind and body communicate is the gut-brain axis. The gut microbiome, which is the community of trillions of bacteria that live in our intestines, plays a vital role in regulating our physical and mental health.

The gut microbiome communicates with the brain through the vagus nerve, a long nerve that connects the gut to the brain. This communication pathway allows the gut microbiome to influence our mood, behavior, and overall well-being.

For example, studies have shown that people with anxiety and depression have different gut microbiomes than people without these conditions. Additionally, probiotics, which are live bacteria that are beneficial to health, have been shown to improve symptoms of anxiety and depression.

The Immune System

The immune system is another important pathway through which the mind and body are connected. When we are stressed, our immune system releases hormones such as cortisol, which can suppress the immune response. This can make us more susceptible to illness and infection.

Conversely, a strong immune system can help to protect us from the negative effects of stress. For example, people who have strong immune systems are less likely to experience anxiety and depression.

The Nervous System

The nervous system is responsible for transmitting messages between the brain and the rest of the body. The sympathetic nervous system is responsible for the "fight-or-flight" response, which is activated when we are stressed. The parasympathetic nervous system is responsible for the "rest-and-digest" response, which is activated when we are relaxed.

When we are stressed, the sympathetic nervous system is activated, which can lead to a number of physical symptoms, such as increased heart rate, sweating, and muscle tension. Over time, chronic stress can lead to wear and tear on the body, increasing the risk of developing chronic health conditions, such as heart disease and diabetes.

The Power of the Mind

While our physical health can have a significant impact on our mental health, the reverse is also true. Our thoughts, beliefs, and emotions can all have a profound impact on our physical well-being.

For example, positive emotions, such as gratitude and optimism, have been shown to boost the immune system and improve overall health. Conversely, negative emotions, such as anger and hostility, have been shown to increase the risk of developing chronic diseases.

The Placebo Effect

The placebo effect is a powerful example of the mind-body connection. The placebo effect is the phenomenon in which a person experiences a beneficial effect from a treatment that is not actually effective. This effect is thought to be due to the power of suggestion and the body's ability to heal itself.

The placebo effect has been shown to be effective in treating a wide range of conditions, including pain, anxiety, and depression. This effect demonstrates the powerful role that the mind can play in healing the body.

Conclusion

The mind and body are inextricably linked, and what affects one inevitably affects the other. By understanding this connection, we can take steps to improve our physical and mental health.

Some simple things that we can do to improve the mind-body connection include:

Eating a healthy diet: A healthy diet is essential for both physical and mental health. Eating plenty of fruits, vegetables, and whole grains can help to improve our overall health and well-being.

Getting regular exercise: Exercise is another great way to improve the mind-body connection. Exercise releases endorphins, which have mood-boosting effects. Exercise can also help to reduce stress and improve sleep quality.

Getting enough sleep: Sleep is essential for both physical and mental health. When we don't get enough sleep, we are more likely to experience anxiety, depression, and other health problems.

Managing stress: Stress is a major contributor to both physical and mental health problems. Learning to manage stress effectively can help to improve our overall health and well-being.

Connecting with others: Social connection is important for both physical and mental health. Spending time with loved ones can help to reduce stress, improve mood, and boost our immune system.

By taking steps to improve the mind-body connection, we can improve our overall health and well-being.

Chapter 3

Holistic Healing: An Overview

Holistic healing is a comprehensive approach to healthcare that addresses the whole person, not just the symptoms of illness. Holistic healers believe that the mind, body, and spirit are interconnected, and that true healing can only occur when all three aspects are in balance.

History of Holistic Healing

Holistic healing practices have been used for centuries in many different cultures around the world. Traditional Chinese medicine, Ayurveda, and Native American medicine are all examples of holistic healing systems that have been used for thousands of years to treat a wide range of illnesses and promote overall well-being.

In recent years, there has been a growing interest in holistic healing in Western countries. This is due in part to the rising dissatisfaction with conventional medicine, which often focuses on treating symptoms rather than addressing the root causes of illness. Holistic healing offers a more comprehensive and patient-centered approach to healthcare that can be effective in treating a wide range of conditions, both physical and mental.

Principles of Holistic Healing

The following are some of the key principles of holistic healing:

The mind, body, and spirit are interconnected and interdependent.

True healing can only occur when all three aspects of the person are in balance.

The body has the ability to heal itself, given the right conditions.

Prevention is better than cure.

The patient is an active participant in their own healing process.

Holistic Healing Practices

There are a wide range of holistic healing practices that can be used to treat a variety of conditions. Some of the most common holistic healing practices include:

Acupuncture

Ayurveda

Chiropractic care

Massage therapy

Naturopathy

Herbal medicine

Yoga

Tai chi

Meditation

Holistic healers typically use a combination of different practices to create individualized treatment plans for their patients.

Benefits of Holistic Healing

Holistic healing offers a number of benefits, including:

Improved physical health: Holistic healing can help to improve physical health by reducing stress, improving sleep, and boosting the immune system. Holistic treatments can also be effective in treating a wide range of physical conditions, from pain and inflammation to digestive problems and chronic diseases.

Improved mental health: Holistic healing can help to improve mental health by reducing anxiety, depression, and stress. Holistic treatments can also be effective in treating a wide range of mental health conditions, from mood disorders to eating disorders and addiction.

Improved spiritual health: Holistic healing can help to improve spiritual health by promoting self-awareness, compassion, and connection to a higher power. Holistic practices can also help us to find meaning and purpose in our lives.

Greater well-being: Holistic healing can help to improve overall well-being by promoting a sense of balance and harmony in our lives. Holistic practices can help us to live more fulfilling and meaningful lives.

Conclusion

Holistic healing is a comprehensive and patient-centered approach to healthcare that can be effective in treating a wide range of conditions, both physical and mental. Holistic healing offers a number of benefits, including improved physical health, improved mental health, improved spiritual health, and greater well-being.

Chapter 4

Mindfulness and Meditation Techniques

Mindfulness and meditation are two powerful tools that can help us to reduce stress, improve our mental health, and live more fulfilling lives. Mindfulness is the practice of paying attention to the present moment without judgment. Meditation is a practice that helps us to train our minds to be more focused and aware.

The Benefits of Mindfulness and Meditation

Mindfulness and meditation have been shown to have a number of benefits, including:

Reduced stress and anxiety:
Mindfulness and meditation can help to reduce stress and anxiety by teaching us to focus on the present moment and let go of worries about the past or future.

Improved mental health: Mindfulness and meditation can help to improve mental health by reducing symptoms of depression, anxiety, and stress. Meditation can also help to improve sleep quality and increase feelings of well-being.

Increased self-awareness: Mindfulness and meditation can help us to become more aware of our thoughts, feelings, and behaviors. This increased self-awareness can help us to make better choices and live more intentional lives.

Improved focus and concentration: Mindfulness and meditation can help to improve focus and concentration by training our minds to be more focused and aware. This improved focus and concentration can benefit us in all areas of our lives, from work and school to relationships and personal hobbies.

Greater compassion and empathy: Mindfulness and meditation can help us to develop greater compassion and empathy for ourselves and others. This increased compassion and empathy can lead to more positive and fulfilling relationships.

How to Practice Mindfulness

There are many different ways to practice mindfulness. Some simple mindfulness exercises include:

Pay attention to your breath: Take a few deep breaths and focus on the sensation of your breath moving in and out of your body. Notice the rise and fall of your chest and abdomen.

Do a body scan: Bring your attention to your body and scan it from head to toe. Notice any sensations that you are experiencing, such as tingling, warmth, or pressure.

Pay attention to your surroundings: Take a few minutes to look around you and notice your surroundings. Pay attention to the sights, sounds, smells, and textures that you experience.

Mindful walking: When you are walking, pay attention to the sensations of your feet on the ground and the movement of your body. Notice the sights, sounds, and smells around you.

How to Practice Meditation

There are many different types of meditation, but most involve sitting in a comfortable position and focusing on your breath or a mantra. Some simple meditation exercises include:

Mindfulness meditation: Sit in a comfortable position and focus on your breath. When your mind wanders, gently bring it back to your breath.

Body scan meditation: Lie down in a comfortable position and bring your attention to your body. Scan your body from head to toe, noticing any sensations that you are experiencing.

Loving-kindness meditation: Sit in a comfortable position and focus on your breath. Bring to mind someone you love and wish them well. Then, extend loving-kindness to all beings, including yourself.

Conclusion

Mindfulness and meditation are powerful tools that can help us to reduce stress, improve our mental health, and live more fulfilling lives. There are many different ways to practice mindfulness and meditation, so find a practice that works for you and make it a regular part of your life.

One-Month Mindfulness and Meditation Plan

Week 1

Focus: Paying attention to the present moment.

Exercises:

Mindful breathing: Sit in a comfortable position and focus on your breath. Notice the rise and fall of your chest and abdomen. If your mind wanders, gently bring it back to your breath.

Body scan meditation: Bring your attention to your body and scan it from head to toe. Notice any sensations that you are experiencing, such as tingling, warmth, or pressure.

Mindful walking: When you are walking, pay attention to the sensations of your feet on the ground and the movement of your body. Notice the sights, sounds, and smells around you.

Week 2

Focus: Cultivating a non-judgmental attitude.

Exercises:

Loving-kindness meditation: Sit in a comfortable position and focus on your breath. Bring to mind someone you love and wish them well. Then, extend loving-kindness to all beings, including yourself.

Gratitude meditation: Take a few minutes each day to reflect on the things you are grateful for. This can be anything from your health to your relationships to the beauty of nature.

Mindful listening: When you are listening to someone, really pay attention to what they are saying. Try to understand their perspective without judgment.

Week 3

Focus: Developing compassion and empathy.

Exercises:

Empathy meditation: Imagine yourself in the shoes of someone who is suffering. Try to understand their pain and offer them compassion.

Metta meditation: Sit in a comfortable position and focus on your breath. Bring to mind someone you care about and wish them well. Then, extend metta (loving-kindness) to all beings, including yourself.

Forgiveness meditation: Take some time to reflect on any grudges or resentments you are holding onto. Try to forgive the people who have wronged you.

Week 4

Focus: Integrating mindfulness and meditation into daily life..

Exercises:

Mindful eating: When you are eating, pay attention to the taste, smell, and texture of your food. Chew slowly and savor each bite.

Mindful driving: When you are driving, pay attention to the sensations of your body in the car and the movement of the vehicle. Notice the sights, sounds, and smells around you.

Mindful working: When you are working, pay attention to the task at hand and try to stay focused on the present moment. Notice any distractions that arise and gently bring your attention back to your work.

Conclusion

This one month mindfulness and meditation plan is a great way to improve your mental health and well-being. By practicing mindfulness and meditation, you can learn to pay attention to the present moment, cultivate a non-judgmental attitude, develop compassion and empathy, and integrate mindfulness into your daily life.

If you have any questions or concerns, please talk to your doctor or a qualified mindfulness and meditation teacher.

Chapter 5

Herbal Remedies for Calmness

In today's fast-paced world, it's more important than ever to find ways to relax and de-stress. Herbal remedies can be a safe and effective way to promote calmness and well-being.

How Herbal Remedies Work

Herbal remedies work by interacting with the body's natural systems. Many herbs contain compounds that have calming and sedative effects. These compounds can help to reduce stress, anxiety, and insomnia.

Choosing the Right Herbal Remedy

There are many different herbal remedies that can be used for calmness. Some of the most popular herbs include:

Chamomile: Chamomile is a gentle herb that has been used for centuries to promote relaxation and sleep. Chamomile is thought to work by binding to benzodiazepine receptors in the brain, which are the same receptors that are targeted by anti-anxiety medications.

Lavender: Lavender is another popular herb that is known for its calming and relaxing effects. Lavender is thought to work by promoting the release of serotonin, a neurotransmitter that is associated with feelings of well-being and relaxation.

Valerian root: Valerian root is a powerful herb that has been shown to be effective in reducing anxiety and improving sleep quality. Valerian root is thought to work by increasing the levels of GABA in the brain, a neurotransmitter that has calming and sedative effects.

Lemon balm: Lemon balm is a member of the mint family that has been shown to have calming and anti-anxiety effects.

Lemon balm is thought to work by inhibiting the breakdown of GABA in the brain, which leads to increased levels of GABA and a calming effect.

Passionflower: Passionflower is a vine that has been used for centuries to promote relaxation and sleep. Passionflower is thought to work by binding to GABA receptors in the brain, which leads to a calming and sedative effect.

How to Use Herbal Remedies

Herbal remedies can be used in a variety of ways, including:

Teas: Herbal teas are a popular way to consume herbal remedies. To make an herbal tea, simply add 1-2 teaspoons of dried herb to a cup of hot water and steep for 5-10 minutes.

Tinctures: Herbal tinctures are concentrated extracts of herbs that are made by soaking the herb in alcohol or vinegar. Tinctures are a convenient way to take herbal remedies, as they can be added to water, juice, or tea.

Capsules: Herbal capsules are a convenient way to take herbal remedies in a pre-measured dose. Herbal capsules are typically made from powdered herb that has been encapsulated in a gelatin or vegetarian capsule.

Dosage

The dosage of an herbal remedy will vary depending on the herb and the form in which it is being taken. It is important to follow the dosage instructions on the product label. If you are unsure about the correct dosage, talk to your doctor or a qualified herbalist.

Safety

Herbal remedies are generally safe when used as directed. However, some herbal remedies can interact with medications, so it is important to talk to your doctor before taking any herbal remedies if you are taking any medications.

Conclusion

Herbal remedies can be a safe and effective way to promote calmness and well-being. If you are looking for a natural way to reduce stress and anxiety, talk to your doctor or a qualified herbalist about which herbal remedies may be right for you.

Additional Information

Other herbs that may be helpful for calmness include: skullcap, hops, kava, and magnolia bark.

It is important to note that some herbal remedies can cause side effects, such as drowsiness, dizziness, and nausea. If you experience any side effects from an herbal remedy, stop taking it and talk to your doctor.

Herbal remedies can be a helpful addition to a healthy lifestyle that includes regular exercise, a healthy diet, and stress-reducing activities such as meditation and yoga.

Chapter 6

The Power of Scent

Smell is one of the most powerful senses when it comes to evoking memories and emotions. Certain scents can instantly transport us back in time to a specific place or event. They can also have a profound effect on our mood and well-being.

Aromatherapy is the practice of using essential oils to promote physical and emotional health. Essential oils are concentrated plant oils that are extracted through distillation or cold pressing. They are highly fragrant and volatile, which means that they can easily be diffused into the air or applied to the skin.

How Aromatherapy Works

Aromatherapy works by stimulating the olfactory bulb, which is located at the back of the nose. The olfactory bulb is connected to the limbic system, which is a complex network of brain structures that is involved in emotion, memory, and behavior.

When we inhale an essential oil, the scent molecules travel through the olfactory bulb to the limbic system. The limbic system then triggers a variety of physiological and emotional responses, depending on the scent.

For example, the scent of lavender has been shown to promote relaxation and sleep, while the scent of rosemary has been shown to improve alertness and concentration.

Benefits of Aromatherapy

Aromatherapy has been shown to have a number of benefits, including:

Reduced stress and anxiety: Aromatherapy can help to reduce stress and anxiety by promoting relaxation and calming the mind.

Improved sleep: Aromatherapy can help to improve sleep quality by promoting relaxation and reducing stress.

Boosted mood: Aromatherapy can help to boost mood by stimulating the release of endorphins, which are hormones that have mood-boosting effects.

Reduced pain: Aromatherapy can help to reduce pain by blocking pain signals in the brain.

Improved cognitive function: Aromatherapy can help to improve cognitive function by stimulating the brain and improving circulation.

How to Use Aromatherapy

There are a number of different ways to use aromatherapy, including:

Diffusion: Diffusion is the most common way to use aromatherapy. Essential oils can be diffused into the air using a diffuser, which is a device that disperses the oil into the air in the form of a fine mist.

Inhalation: Essential oils can also be inhaled directly from the bottle or from a tissue.

Topical application: Essential oils can be diluted in a carrier oil, such as jojoba oil or coconut oil, and applied to the skin.

Choosing the Right Essential Oils

There are many different essential oils available, each with its own unique scent and properties. When choosing essential oils for aromatherapy, it is important to consider your individual needs and preferences.

Some of the most popular essential oils for aromatherapy include:

Lavender: Lavender is a calming and relaxing oil that is often used to promote sleep and reduce stress.

Peppermint: Peppermint is an invigorating and stimulating oil that is often used to improve alertness and concentration.

Eucalyptus: Eucalyptus is a decongestant and expectorant oil that is often used to relieve respiratory problems.

Tea tree oil: Tea tree oil is an antibacterial and antifungal oil that is often used to treat skin problems.

Lemon: Lemon is a refreshing and uplifting oil that is often used to boost mood and improve cognitive function.

Dosage

The dosage of essential oils will vary depending on the method of application. It is important to follow the directions on the product label. If you are unsure about the correct dosage, talk to your doctor or a qualified aromatherapist.

Safety

Essential oils are generally safe when used as directed. However, some essential oils can be toxic if ingested or applied to the skin undiluted. It is important to read the product label carefully before using any essential oils and to follow the directions for safe use.

Conclusion

Aromatherapy is a safe and effective way to promote physical and emotional health. By using essential oils to stimulate the sense of smell, aromatherapy can help to reduce stress, improve sleep, boost mood, reduce pain, and improve cognitive function.

If you are looking for a natural way to improve your health and well-being, aromatherapy is a great option to consider.

One Month Aromatherapy Plan

Week 1

Focus: Relaxation and stress relief.

Essential oils: Lavender, chamomile, bergamot, ylang-ylang.

How to use: Diffuse the essential oils in your home or office, or add a few drops to your bathwater. You can also apply the essential oils to your skin, diluted in a carrier oil such as jojoba oil or coconut oil.

Week 2

Focus: Energy and focus.

Essential oils: Peppermint, rosemary, lemon, grapefruit.

How to use: Diffuse the essential oils in your home or office, or inhale them directly from the bottle. You can also add a few drops of the essential oils to your shampoo or conditioner.

Week 3

Focus: Sleep and insomnia.

Essential oils: Lavender, chamomile, valerian root, vetiver.

How to use: Diffuse the essential oils in your bedroom at night, or add a few drops to your pillowcase. You can also take a warm bath with the essential oils added to the water.

Week 4

Focus: Pain relief.

Essential oils: Peppermint, eucalyptus, lavender, rosemary.

How to use: Dilute the essential oils in a carrier oil and apply to the affected area. You can also diffuse the essential oils in your home or office.

This one month aromatherapy plan is a great way to improve your health and well-being. By using essential oils to stimulate your sense of smell, aromatherapy can help to reduce stress, improve sleep, boost mood, reduce pain, and improve cognitive function.

If you have any questions or concerns, please talk to your doctor or a qualified aromatherapist.

Chapter 7

Healing Through Nutrition

The food we eat has a profound impact on our physical and mental health. Eating a healthy diet can help us to maintain a healthy weight, reduce our risk of chronic diseases, and improve our overall well-being.

Nutritional therapy is a type of alternative medicine that uses diet to promote healing and prevent disease. Nutritional therapists believe that by eating a nutrient-rich diet, we can support our body's natural healing processes and improve our overall health.

How Nutritional Therapy Works

Nutritional therapy works by providing the body with the nutrients it needs to function properly. These nutrients include vitamins, minerals, antioxidants, and other essential compounds.

When we eat a healthy diet, our bodies are able to repair themselves and fight off infection. We also have more energy and vitality.

Nutritional therapy can be used to treat a wide range of conditions, including:

Digestive problems

Skin problems

Weight problems

Fatigue

Anxiety

Depression

The Benefits of Nutritional Therapy

Nutritional therapy offers a number of benefits, including:

Improved physical health: Nutritional therapy can help to improve physical health by providing the body with the nutrients it needs to function properly. This can lead to improved digestion, weight loss, and reduced risk of chronic diseases.

Improved mental health: Nutritional therapy can also help to improve mental health by reducing inflammation and supporting the production of neurotransmitters. This can lead to reduced anxiety, depression, and improved cognitive function.

Increased energy and vitality: Eating a healthy diet can help to increase energy and vitality. This is because the body is able to use the nutrients in food to fuel its activities.

Reduced risk of chronic diseases:
Eating a healthy diet can help to reduce the risk of chronic diseases, such as heart disease, stroke, cancer, and diabetes. This is because a healthy diet provides the body with the nutrients it needs to protect itself from disease.

How to Find a Qualified Nutritional Therapist

If you are interested in nutritional therapy, it is important to find a qualified nutritional therapist. A qualified nutritional therapist will have the training and experience to help you develop a personalized nutrition plan that meets your individual needs.

To find a qualified nutritional therapist, you can ask your doctor for a referral or search online for a nutritional therapist in your area. You can also look for nutritional therapists who are certified by a professional organization, such as the American Association of Nutritional Consultants (AANC) or the National Association of Nutritional Professionals (NANP).

Conclusion

Nutritional therapy is a safe and effective way to improve your health and well-being. By eating a healthy diet, you can provide your body with the nutrients it needs to heal itself and thrive.

If you are interested in learning more about nutritional therapy, I encourage you to talk to your doctor or a qualified nutritional therapist. They can help you to develop a personalized nutrition plan that meets your individual needs and helps you to achieve your health goals.

One Month Nutritional Therapy Plan

Week 1

Focus: Detoxification and elimination.

Goals: To cleanse the body of toxins and promote elimination.

Foods to eat: Fruits, vegetables, whole grains, legumes, lean protein.

Foods to avoid: Processed foods, sugary drinks, unhealthy fats, red meat.

Sample Meal Plan:

Breakfast: Oatmeal with berries and nuts.

Lunch: Salad with grilled chicken or fish.

Dinner: Lentil soup with whole-grain bread.

Snacks: Fruits, vegetables, nuts, seeds.

Week 2

Focus: Nutrient replenishment.

Goals: To replenish the body with essential nutrients.

Foods to eat: Fruits, vegetables, whole grains, legumes, lean protein, healthy fats.

Foods to avoid: Processed foods, sugary drinks, unhealthy fats, red meat.

Sample Meal Plan

Breakfast: Yogurt with fruit and granola.

Lunch: Sandwich on whole-grain bread with lean protein, vegetables, and hummus.

Dinner: Salmon with roasted vegetables and brown rice

Snacks: Trail mix, smoothies, vegetable sticks.

Week 3

Focus: Digestion and gut health.

Goals: To improve digestion and support gut health.

Foods to eat: Fermented foods, probiotics, prebiotics, fiber.

Foods to avoid: Processed foods, sugary drinks, unhealthy fats, red meat.

Sample Meal Plan

Breakfast: Kefir smoothie with fruit and spinach.

Lunch: Salad with grilled chicken or fish, vegetables, and beans.

Dinner: Chicken stir-fry with brown rice.

Snacks: Yogurt, kimchi, sauerkraut.

Week 4

Focus: Maintenance and lifestyle changes.

Goals: To maintain the progress made in the previous three weeks and make lasting lifestyle changes.

Foods to eat: A variety of nutrient-rich foods from all food groups.

Foods to avoid: Processed foods, sugary drinks, unhealthy fats, red meat.

Sample Meal Plan

Breakfast: Eggs with whole-grain toast and avocado.

Lunch: Leftover chicken stir-fry.

Dinner: Grilled salmon with roasted vegetables and quinoa.

Snacks: Fruits, vegetables, nuts, seeds.

Tips for Success

Set realistic goals: Don't try to change too much too soon. Start by making small changes to your diet and gradually add more as you become more comfortable.

Focus on whole, unprocessed foods: Whole foods are packed with nutrients and fiber, which are essential for good health.

Cook more meals at home: This gives you more control over the ingredients in your food and helps you to avoid processed foods.

Drink plenty of water: Water is essential for good health and can help to flush toxins from the body.

Be patient and consistent: It takes time to make lasting changes to your diet. Be patient with yourself and don't give up if you slip up from time to time.

This one month nutritional therapy plan is a great way to improve your health and well-being. By following the plan, you can detoxify your body, replenish your nutrients, improve your digestion, and make lasting lifestyle changes.

If you have any questions or concerns, please talk to your doctor or a qualified nutritional therapist.

Chapter 8
Yoga and Tai Chi for Balance

Balance is an essential component of everyday life. It allows us to walk, run, and perform other basic tasks without falling over. It also helps us to maintain our posture and avoid injuries.

There are a number of factors that can affect our balance, including our age, fitness level, and neurological health.

However, there are also a number of things we can do to improve our balance, such as practicing yoga or tai chi.

Yoga

Yoga is an ancient practice that originated in India over 5,000 years ago. It is a mind-body practice that combines physical postures, breathing exercises, and meditation. Yoga is often used to improve flexibility, strength, and balance, but it can also be beneficial for mental health and well-being.

How Yoga Improves Balance

Yoga improves balance by strengthening the muscles around the joints, improving flexibility, and increasing body awareness.

Strengthening the muscles around the joints: Many yoga poses require you to balance on one leg or in an inverted position. This helps to strengthen the muscles around the ankles, knees, and hips, which are essential for maintaining balance.

Improving flexibility: Yoga also helps to improve flexibility, which is important for balance. When your muscles are flexible, you are less likely to lose your balance when you move or change positions.

Increasing body awareness: Yoga also helps to increase body awareness. This means that you are more aware of where your body is in space and how it is moving. This increased body awareness can help you to maintain your balance even in challenging situations.

Tai Chi

Tai Chi is a chinese martial art that is often practiced for its health benefits. Tai chi is a gentle, low-impact exercise that combines slow, flowing movements with deep breathing. Tai Chi is often used to improve balance, flexibility, and strength, but it can also be beneficial for mental health and well-being.

How Tai Chi Improves Balance

Tai Chi improves balance by strengthening the muscles around the joints, improving flexibility, and increasing body awareness.

Strengthening the muscles around the joints: Many Tai Chi movements require you to balance on one leg or in an inverted position. This helps to strengthen the muscles around the ankles, knees, and hips, which are essential for maintaining balance.

Improving flexibility: Tai Chi also helps to improve flexibility, which is important for balance. When your muscles are flexible, you are less likely to lose your balance when you move or change positions.

Increasing body awareness: Tai Chi also helps to increase body awareness. This means that you are more aware of where your body is in space and how it is moving. This increased body awareness can help you to maintain your balance even in challenging situations.

Conclusion

Yoga and Tai Chi are both excellent practices for improving balance. Yoga is a more physically demanding practice, while Tai Chi is a more gentle practice. Both Yoga and Tai Chi can be beneficial for people of all ages and fitness levels.

If you are interested in improving your balance, I encourage you to try Yoga or Tai Chi. Both practices can help you to strengthen your muscles, improve your flexibility, and increase your body awareness. With regular practice, you will notice a significant improvement in your balance.

Additional Information

Other activities that can help to improve balance include: walking, swimming, and dancing.

It is important to talk to your doctor before starting any new exercise program, especially if you have any health concerns.

If you experience any pain or discomfort while practicing Yoga or Tai Chi, stop and consult with your doctor or a qualified instructor.

Benefits of Yoga and Tai Chi

In addition to improving balance, Yoga and Tai Chi offer a number of other benefits, including:

Reduced stress and anxiety

Improved sleep quality

Increased energy levels

Reduced pain and stiffness

Improved cardiovascular health

Enhanced mental clarity and focus

If you are looking for a way to improve your overall health and well-being, Yoga and Tai Chi are both excellent options to consider.

One Month Yoga Plan

Week 1

Focus: Building a foundation.

Poses: Mountain pose, tree pose, downward-facing dog, plank pose, child's pose.

Sequence

Mountain pose (5 breaths).

Tree pose (5 breaths on each side).

Downward-facing dog (5 breaths).

Plank pose (30 seconds).

Child's pose (5 breaths).

Repeat: 2-3 times.

Week 2

Focus: Sun salutations.

Poses: Sun salutation A, sun salutation B.

Sequence

Sun salutation A (5 rounds).

Sun salutation B (3 rounds).

Repeat: 2-3 times.

Week 3

Focus: Standing poses.

Poses: Warrior I, warrior II, triangle pose, extended side angle pose.

Sequence

Warrior I (5 breaths on each side).

Warrior II (5 breaths on each side).

Triangle pose (5 breaths on each side).

Extended side angle pose (5 breaths on each side).

Repeat: 2-3 times.

Week 4

Focus: Seated and supine poses.

Poses: Seated forward fold, seated twist, corpse pose.

Sequence

Seated forward fold (5 breaths).

Seated twist (5 breaths on each side).

Corpse pose (5 minutes).

Repeat: 2-3 times.

Tips for Success

Find a qualified instructor: It is important to find a qualified instructor who can teach you the proper techniques and ensure that you are practicing safely.

Start slowly: Don't try to do too much too soon. Start with a few simple poses and gradually increase the difficulty as you become more comfortable.

Be consistent: The key to success with yoga is consistency. Try to practice for at least 10 minutes each day.

Be patient: It takes time to develop flexibility and strength. Don't get discouraged if you don't see results immediately. Just keep practicing and you will eventually see the benefits.

Conclusion

This one month yoga plan is a great way to improve your flexibility, strength, and balance. Yoga is a safe and effective practice that can be beneficial for people of all ages and fitness levels.

If you have any questions or concerns, please talk to your doctor or a qualified yoga instructor.

One Month Tai Chi Plan

Week 1

Focus: Learning the basic movements.

Moves: Ward off, roll back, press, push.

Sequence

Ward off (5 repetitions on each side).

Roll back (5 repetitions on each side).

Press (5 repetitions on each side).

Push (5 repetitions on each side).

Repeat: 2-3 times

Week 2

Focus: Putting the movements together

Moves: Ward off, roll back, press, push, cloud hands

Sequence

Ward off (5 repetitions on each side).

Roll back (5 repetitions on each side).

Press (5 repetitions on each side).

Push (5 repetitions on each side).

Cloud hands (5 repetitions on each side).

Repeat: 2-3 times.

Week 3

Focus: Refining the movements.

Moves: Ward off, roll back, press, push, cloud hands, single whip.

Sequence

Ward off (5 repetitions on each side).

Roll back (5 repetitions on each side).

Press (5 repetitions on each side).

Push (5 repetitions on each side).

Cloud hands (5 repetitions on each side).

Single whip (5 repetitions on each side).

Repeat: 2-3 times.

Week 4

Focus: Putting it all together.

Moves: Ward off, roll back, press, push, cloud hands, single whip, brush knee, side kick.

Sequence

Ward off (5 repetitions on each side).

Roll back (5 repetitions on each side).

Press (5 repetitions on each side).

Push (5 repetitions on each side).

Cloud hands (5 repetitions on each side).

Single whip (5 repetitions on each side).

Brush knee (5 repetitions on each side).

Side kick (5 repetitions on each side).

Repeat: 2-3 times.

Tips for Success

Find a qualified instructor: It is important to find a qualified instructor who can teach you the proper techniques and ensure that you are practicing safely.

Start slowly: Don't try to do too much too soon. Start with a few simple moves and gradually increase the difficulty as you become more comfortable.

Be consistent: The key to success with tai chi is consistency. Try to practice for at least 10 minutes each day.

Be patient: It takes time to develop the coordination and balance required for tai chi. Don't get discouraged if you don't see results immediately. Just keep practicing and you will eventually see the benefits.

Conclusion

This one month Tai Chi plan is a great way to improve your balance, flexibility, and strength. Tai Chi is a safe and effective practice that can be beneficial for people of all ages and fitness levels.

If you have any questions or concerns, please talk to your doctor or a qualified Tai Chi instructor.

Chapter 9

Creating a Tranquil Environment

In today's fast-paced world, it's more important than ever to create a tranquil environment at home. A tranquil environment can help to reduce stress, improve sleep, and boost overall well-being.

There are many different ways to create a tranquil environment, and what works for one person may not work for another. However, there are some general principles that can be applied to any space.

Declutter and Organize

One of the best ways to create a tranquil environment is to declutter and organize your space. When your home is cluttered, it can be difficult to relax and de-stress. Take some time to go through your belongings and get rid of anything you don't need. Once you have decluttered, take some time to organize your belongings so that everything has a place.

Choose Calming Colors

The colors you choose for your home can have a big impact on the atmosphere. Calming colors, such as blue, green, and lavender, can help to create a more tranquil environment. Avoid using bright or harsh colors, as these can be stimulating and stressful.

Add Natural Elements

Bringing the outdoors in is a great way to create a more tranquil environment. Add plants to your home, or place fresh flowers in a vase. You can also use natural materials, such as wood and stone, in your décor.

Create a Cozy Atmosphere

A cozy atmosphere can be very calming and inviting. Add soft throws and pillows to your furniture, and use warm lighting to create a cozy ambiance. You can also add scented candles or an essential oil diffuser to your space.

Reduce Noise

Noise can be a major source of stress. If you live in a noisy area, try to find ways to reduce the noise levels in your home.

You can use white noise machines, earplugs, or soundproofing materials.

Create a Relaxing Space

Set aside a special place in your home where you can relax and de-stress. This could be a reading nook, a meditation room, or simply a comfortable chair in a quiet corner. Make sure your relaxation space is free from distractions and that it is a place where you feel comfortable and at peace.

Conclusion

Creating a tranquil environment at home is essential for reducing stress, improving sleep, and boosting overall well-being. By following the tips in this chapter, you can create a space that is calming, inviting, and restorative.

Here are some additional tips for creating a tranquil environment:

Take some time for yourself each day to relax and de-stress. This could involve reading, taking a bath, or listening to calming music.

Make sure your bedroom is dark, quiet, and cool. These conditions are ideal for sleep.

Avoid watching TV or working in bed. This can make it difficult to relax and fall asleep.

Create a regular sleep routine and stick to it as much as possible. This will help to regulate your body's natural sleep-wake cycle.

Talk to your doctor if you're having trouble sleeping. There may be an underlying medical condition that is causing your insomnia.

Chapter 10

Self-Care Practices for Daily Wellness

In today's fast-paced world, it's more important than ever to make time for self-care. Self-care is anything you do to take care of your physical, emotional, and mental health. It can include activities such as exercise, healthy eating, getting enough sleep, and spending time with loved ones.

Self-care is not selfish. It's essential for your overall well-being. When you take care of yourself, you are better able to take care of others.

There are many different ways to practice self-care. The aim is to find activities that you enjoy and that fit into your lifestyle. Here are a few ideas:

Physical self-care

Exercise regularly. Aim for at least 30 minutes of moderate-intense exercise most days of the week. Eat a healthy diet. Choose plenty of fruits, vegetables, and whole grains. Limit processed foods, sugary drinks, and unhealthy fats.

Get enough sleep. Most adults need 7-8 hours of sleep per night.

Emotional self-care

Spend time with loved ones. Connect with friends and family on a regular basis.

Do things that you enjoy. Make time for activities that bring you joy, such as reading, listening to music, or spending time in nature.

Learn to say no. It's okay to say no to things that you don't want to do. Don't overcommit yourself.

Mental self-care

Practice mindfulness: Mindfulness is the practice of paying attention to the present moment without judgment. There are many different ways to practice mindfulness, such as meditation, Yoga, and Tai Chi.

Challenge negative thoughts: When you find yourself thinking negative thoughts, challenge them. Ask yourself if there is any evidence to support your thoughts. Ask if you are being fair to yourself?

Set realistic goals: Don't set yourself up for failure by setting unrealistic goals. Break down your goals into smaller, more manageable steps.

Self-care is an ongoing journey: It is not something that you can do perfectly overnight. There will be times when you slip up. That is okay. Just pick yourself up and keep going.

The most important thing is to be kind to yourself. Treat yourself with the same compassion and understanding that you would offer a friend.

Benefits of Self-Care

There are many benefits to practicing self-care, including:

Reduced stress and anxiety

Improved sleep

Increased energy and vitality

Stronger immune system

Improved mood

Increased self-confidence

Better relationships

Greater sense of purpose and fulfillment

Conclusion

Self-care is essential for your overall health and well-being. By taking care of yourself, you are better able to take care of others.

Make time for self-care every day. Even small acts of self-care can make a big difference in your life.

Chapter 11

Embracing Change and Growth

Change is a constant in life. It can be positive or negative, expected or unexpected. But one thing is for sure: change is inevitable.

How we respond to change can make all the difference in our lives. We can either resist change and suffer, or we can embrace change and grow.

Embracing change means accepting that change is a part of life and that it can be a positive force. It means being open to new experiences and challenges, and being willing to learn and grow.

It is not always easy to embrace change. Sometimes it can be scary or uncomfortable. But if we can learn to embrace change, we will be better equipped to handle whatever life throws our way.

Here are a few tips for embracing change

Be open to new experiences: Don't be afraid to try new things, even if they are outside of your comfort zone. You never know what you might discover about yourself.

Challenge your negative thoughts: When you find yourself thinking negative thoughts about change, challenge them. Ask yourself if there is any evidence to support your thoughts. Are you being fair to yourself?

Focus on the positive: When you are faced with change, try to focus on the positive aspects. What are the opportunities that this change could bring? How could this change help you to grow?

Take small steps: If you are feeling overwhelmed by change, don't try to do too much at once. Break down your goals into smaller, more manageable steps.

Be patient with yourself: Embracing change takes time. Don't be hard on yourself if you don't change overnight. Just keep practicing and you will eventually get there.

Benefits of Embracing Change

There are many benefits to embracing change, including:

Reduced stress and anxiety: When we resist change, we create stress and anxiety for ourselves. But when we embrace change, we can reduce our stress levels and live more peacefully.

Increased resilience: When we embrace change, we become more resilient. We learn to adapt to new situations and to bounce back from setbacks.

Greater creativity and innovation: Change can spark creativity and innovation. When we are open to new ideas and experiences, we are more likely to come up with new and innovative solutions to problems.

Personal growth: Change can help us to grow as individuals. When we step outside of our comfort zones, we learn new things about ourselves and we become more confident and capable.

Conclusion

Change is a part of life. We can either resist change and suffer, or we can embrace change and grow.

If we can learn to embrace change, we will be better equipped to handle whatever life throws our way. We will be more resilient, more creative, and more fulfilled.

Here are some additional tips for embracing change:

Talk to someone you trust: If you are struggling to embrace change, talk to a friend, family member, or therapist. They can offer support and guidance.

Read books and articles about change: There are many helpful books and articles available about how to embrace change. Reading about the experiences of others can help you to feel less alone.

Attend workshops or seminars on change: There are many workshops and seminars available that can help you to learn how to embrace change. These workshops can provide you with tools and techniques for dealing with change in a positive way.

Embracing change is not always easy, but it is worth it. When we embrace change, we open ourselves up to new possibilities and experiences. We

become more resilient, more creative,
and more fulfilled.

Epilogue

Finding Your Path to Serenity

In today's fast-paced world, it can be difficult to find serenity. We are constantly bombarded with information and stimuli, and it can be hard to find a moment to relax and de-stress.

But serenity is essential for our well-being. It is a state of inner peace and calm that allows us to cope with the challenges of life with greater ease.

There is no one-size-fits-all path to serenity. What works for one person may not work for another. But there are some general principles that can help you to find your own path to serenity.

Here are a few tips:

Identify your sources of stress: Once you know what is causing you stress, you can start to develop strategies for managing it.

Make time for yourself: Even if it is just for a few minutes each day, make time for yourself to do something you enjoy. This could be reading, listening to music, or spending time in nature.

Learn to say no: It is okay to say no to things that you don't want to do. Don't overcommit yourself.

Set realistic goals: When you set unrealistic goals, you're setting yourself up for failure. Break down your goals into smaller, more manageable steps.

Be kind to yourself: Forgive yourself for your mistakes and don't be too hard on yourself. Everyone makes mistakes.

Practice mindfulness: Mindfulness is the practice of paying attention to the present moment without judgment. There are many different ways to practice mindfulness, such as meditation, Yoga, and Tai Chi.

Connect with nature: Spending time in nature has been shown to reduce stress and improve mood. Try to spend some time in nature every day, even if it is just for a few minutes.

Help others: Helping others can make you feel good about yourself and can also help to reduce stress. Volunteer your time or donate to a cause that you care about.

Finding your path to serenity is a journey. It takes time and effort. But it is worth it. When you find serenity, you will be better able to cope with the challenges of life and live a more fulfilling life.

Conclusion

Serenity is a state of inner peace and calm that allows us to cope with the challenges of life with greater ease. There is no one-size-fits-all path to serenity, but there are some general principles that can help you to find your own path.

By following the tips in this chapter, you can start to create a more serene life for yourself.

Here are some additional tips for finding your path to serenity:

Be patient with yourself: Finding serenity takes time and effort. Don't get discouraged if you don't see results immediately. Just keep practicing and you will eventually get there.

Talk to someone you trust: If you are struggling to find serenity, talk to a friend, family member, or therapist. They can offer support and guidance.

Read books and articles about serenity: There are many helpful books and articles available about how to find serenity. Reading about the experiences of others can help you to feel less alone.

Attend workshops or seminars on serenity: There are many workshops and seminars available that can help you to learn how to find serenity. These workshops can provide you with tools and techniques for creating a more serene life.

Finding serenity is not always easy, but it is worth it. When you find serenity, you will be better able to cope with the challenges of life and live a more fulfilling life.